All
About
Pneumonia

Symptoms, Causes, Types, Stages & Treatment

Dr. Sheila Harrison

Disclaimer

This content serves to provide general information about the disease and aims to empower you to seek prompt medical assistance if necessary to prevent complications. It's essential to stress that this information is not a substitute for consulting a qualified physician. The field of medical science is continually evolving, and due to the dynamic nature of medical knowledge, we recommend seeking expert advice if you encounter any inconsistencies or intend to take action based on the information in this content. Never disregard professional medical guidance or delay treatment based on something you've read online, including this material, or from any other online source. Always remember that the internet cannot cure you; rather, healing comes through the guidance of medical professionals and the providence of God.

Table of Content

Section 1

How Our Lungs Work

The main function of our lungs is to get carbon dioxide out of our bloodstream so that we can breathe it out as a waste product, and to get oxygen – the chemical essential for the health of every part of our body – from the air into our bloodstream.

When we breathe, we draw in air through our nose and mouth. This air travels down our trachea or windpipe and into our lungs. The airways continue to branch off into each lobe, and then into further, smaller branches. At the end of each of the smallest branches are bundles of air sacs, called alveoli. The alveoli are surrounded by a network of fine blood vessels. Blood that has delivered oxygen all around the body returns to the heart depleted of nutrients and is pumped into the fine vessels in the tissues of the lungs. It can then excrete carbon dioxide, and pick up oxygen then return to the heart where the oxygen-rich blood can be pumped around the body again. This cycle continues throughout our lives with every heartbeat. With every breath, we take in microbes – bacteria, viruses and fungal spores.

Thankfully, our lungs have several lines of defence to ensure that these microbes don't cause any serious problems. Some get stuck in the moisture and mucous of our nose and mouth and are filtered through the fine hairs inside our noses. Microscopic cells in the lining of our respiratory system then push these particles out of the system. Our lungs are also lined with fine mucous which act as a protective barrier and the immune system provides cells which identify and destroy any microbes that enter.

Sometimes, however, our body's natural defence system is not enough. Certain microbes are particularly good at crossing those barriers. Some health conditions may also weaken our defence system and make it easier for this to happen. When there are enough microbes colonising our lung tissue, they start to affect our lung function. Our immune system responds, filling our tissues with fluids and the fighter cells of the immune system. This causes swelling or inflammation, restricting the amount of tissue that can be used for gas exchange.

When we have reduced lung function, our body finds it harder to get enough oxygen and to blow off enough carbon dioxide. Our bodies automatically try to compensate for this by increasing the heart rate and by breathing harder and faster. If our lung function is seriously impaired, we can develop a build-up of carbon dioxide in the body which develops into a condition called acidosis, where our blood is literally more acidic than is healthy. Our kidneys will then try to compensate for this, which then affects the function of every essential organ in the body. This systemic, whole-body, response is known as sepsis and can be deadly.

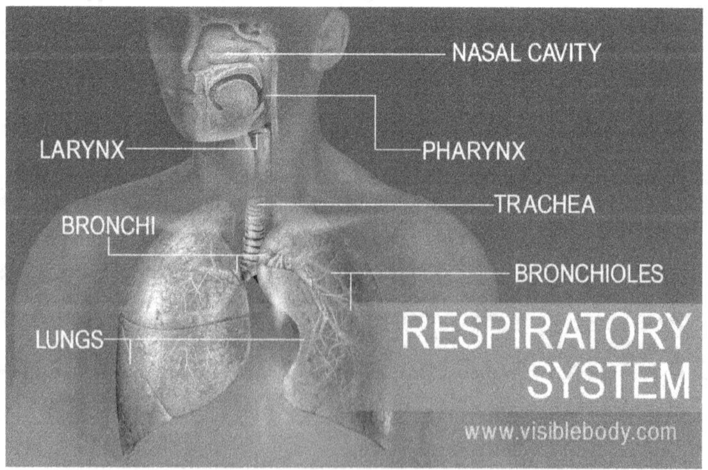

Section 2

What is pneumonia?

Pneumonia is an infection in our lung or lungs which causes swelling of the delicate tissues of the lung. We may also talk about people having a 'chest infection' or lower respiratory tract infection ('LRTI'), either of which may be pneumonia.Pneumonia is a lung disease that causes the air sacs in one or both lungs to become inflamed. Cough with pus, fever, chills, and trouble breathing can result and the air sacs accumulate with fluid or pus. Different kinds of microbes, including bacteria, viruses, and fungus can cause pneumonia.

Swelling of the delicate tissues of the lung

The severity of this condition can be from minor to life-threatening and sometimes death occurs. Infants and young children and individuals over the age of 65, and people with health issues or weak immune systems are at greater risk. The most common type of pneumonia, bacterial pneumonia, is more serious than other types, with symptoms that need medical attention. Bacterial pneumonia symptoms can result gradually or unexpectedly. Fever can be of dangerously high temperatures of 105 degrees Fahrenheit, with excessive sweating and fast breathing and heart rate may also increase.

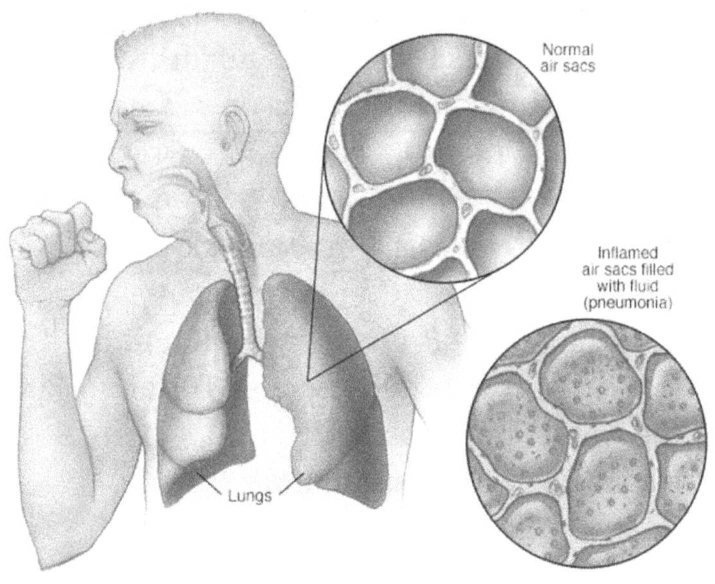

Due to deficiency of oxygen in the blood, the lips and nail beds may become bluish. The mental condition of a patient might be confused or changed. The symptoms of viral pneumonia usually appear in a few days after the infection. The symptoms mostly worsen within a day or two, with an increasing cough and shortness of breath.

Pneumonia can become serious and can cause life-threatening complications such as sepsis or abscesses in the lung. Pneumonia may be caused by a virus, bacteria, occasionally a fungus. The body's immune response to an infection causes inflammation of the tissues of the alveoli – the tiny sacs in the lungs where the gases are exchanged.

The elderly *(alongside young children)* are the most susceptible to it. This may be due to underlying health problems or weakened immune systems.

To understand pneumonia, it helps to understand how our lungs work.

Section 3

What causes pneumonia?

Pneumonia is an infection caused by a microbe or 'germ.

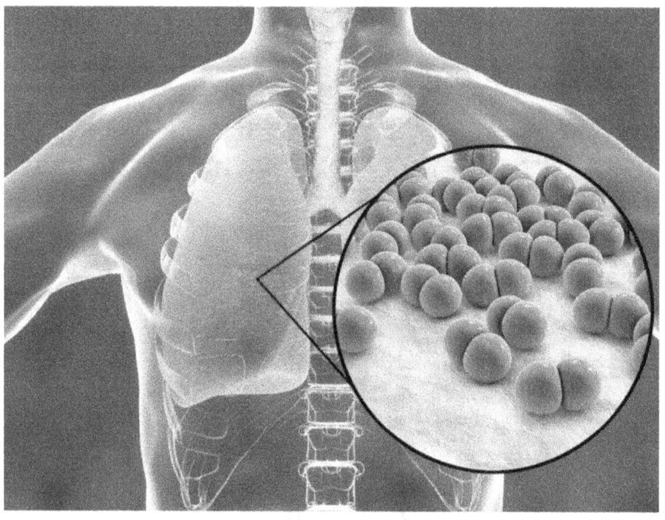

The air sacs might eventually fill up with pus and liquids as a result of the inflammation, resulting in pneumonia symptoms. Streptococcus pneumonia is the most prevalent cause of bacterial pneumonia.

This microbe can be:

- **Bacterial:** There are several types of bacteria that can cause pneumonia. Most community-acquired pneumonia and all aspiration pneumonia are caused by bacteria. Bacterial pneumonia can usually be well treated with a course of antibiotics.

- **Viral:** The most common type of virus that causes pneumonia in adults is the influenza virus or 'flu'. Viruses are not affected by antibiotics. In children, pneumonia is commonly caused by a virus called 'RSV'.

- **Fungal:** Pneumonia can also develop from an infection caught by breathing in the spores of certain types of fungus. This is less common, but when it does occur, it tends to happen in people who already have a compromised immune system.

Other causes of the condition include:

- **Mycoplasma pneumoniae:** *Mycoplasma pneumoniae* bacteria commonly cause mild infections of the respiratory system (the parts of the body involved in breathing). Sometimes these bacteria can cause more serious lung infections that require care in a hospital. Good hygiene is important to help decrease the spread of *M. pneumoniae* and other respiratory germs.

- **Haemophilus influenzae:** Haemophilus influenzae disease is a name for any illness caused by bacteria called H. influenzae. Some of these illnesses, like ear infections, are mild while others, like bloodstream infections, are very serious. In spite of the name, H. influenzae does not cause influenza (the flu). Vaccines can prevent one type of H. influenzae (type b or Hib) disease.

- **Legionella pneumophila:** Legionella bacteria can cause a serious type of pneumonia (lung infection) called Legionnaires' disease. Legionella bacteria can also cause a less serious illness called Pontiac fever.

- Infection with the human parainfluenza virus (HPIV) and the human metapneumovirus (HMPV) infection

- Chickenpox, measles increase risk

- Infection with the adenovirus

- Infection with a coronavirus

Section 4

Is pneumonia contagious?

The microbes that cause pneumonia can be passed from person to person, especially those that cause viral pneumonia. Some microbes can be passed from other animals to humans as well. Bacteria can also be introduced to the lungs when someone accidentally inhales food or fluids. These microbes can cause lung infections.

However, it is important to note that exposure to the microbes that may cause pneumonia does not necessarily mean that you will get ill, and if you do get ill, it may not necessarily become pneumonia. Sometimes our natural immune response can prevent infectious microbes from causing serious problems, but other times infections can become severe. The combination of a serious infection and our own immune system's response to it is what causes pneumonia.

People most at risk of infections and complications should take extra care to avoid people or situations where they will be exposed to the microbes that cause infections. As the bugs that cause pneumonia are contagious, people living in close quarters are at higher risk of having pneumonia. This includes people living in military barracks, student accommodation, and in care homes. People in care homes are also more likely to have other risk factors.

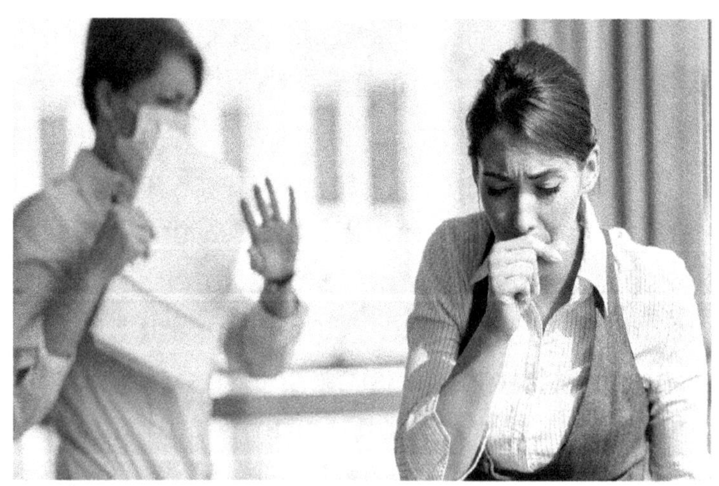

Section 5

Symptoms of Pneumonia

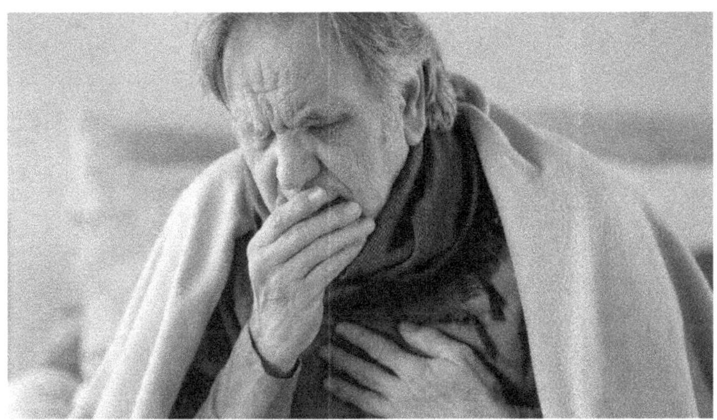

The signs of pneumonia in older adults may be different compared to other age groups.

As such, these are some of the possible symptoms one may experience.

- Feeling weak or dizzy, which may cause a person to fall
- Do not have a fever or a significant body temperature change
- Experience confusion

- Change in the ability to perform daily activities
- Experience difficulty in urinating
- Undergo a lack of appetite
- Worsening of existing health conditions

As these signs may not seem obvious as pneumonia, some older adults get diagnosed later, worsening the condition at hand.

The usual symptoms of pneumonia may also be experienced, however:

- Coughing that produces phlegm is one of them (mucus)
- Fever, sweating, or chills are all symptoms.
- Chest discomfort that gets worse when you breathe or cough
- Tedness - Emotions of exhaustion or weariness
- Shortness of breath that occurs when doing typical activities or even while resting
- Rapid breathing

- Infants may appear to be symptom-free, yet they may vomit, be tired, or have difficulty drinking or eating.
- Children under the age of five may have rapid breathing or wheezing.

When to See a Doctor

As pneumonia can worsen quickly in higher-risk groups such as young children and the elderly, it is necessary to detect the condition as soon as possible.

Some of these signs may require immediate attention:

- Breathing difficulties
- Bluish hue to your face, nails or lips
- Chest pains
- Abnormal body temperature *(significantly lower or higher than usual)*
- Changes in functional status

Before experiencing such emergencies, it is vital to identify the closest clinic or hospital, before the time of need. This will assist in last-minute logistics that can potentially save one's life.

Section 6

Types of Pneumonia

There are several ways of describing pneumonia; we may talk about the areas of the lungs affected and the type of microbe that caused the infection. We may also talk about the way a person acquired pneumonia, which tells us a lot about the kind of microbe that may have caused it and the kind of path the illness may take.

Here are some of the common types of pneumonia:

- **Community-Acquired Pneumonia:** This refers to pneumonia that started in the community and not in a hospital or institutional setting.

- **Hospital-Acquired Pneumonia:** This refers to pneumonia which developed in a hospital, secondary to the reason for admission. It also has to be at least 48 hours after admission, as pneumonia which develops within 48 hours is most likely to come from a microbe caught in the community. People in hospitals are usually in close proximity to other people who are unwell and may have a compromised immune system due to existing illnesses. Hence, they may be more exposed to certain sorts of viruses and bacteria while in the hospital, including some which are harder to treat with antibiotics.

- **Ventilator-Acquired Pneumonia:** Also referred to as ventilator-associated pneumonia, ventilator-acquired pneumonia is a type of hospital-acquired pneumonia which occurs when people are intubated and mechanically ventilated in a hospital's intensive care unit. This means they have a tube in their throat attached to a machine which helps them to breathe or breathes for them. People on ventilators in intensive care are already unwell and so developing ventilator acquired pneumonia as a secondary complication can be highly dangerous.

- **Aspiration Pneumonia:** This is a type of pneumonia developed as a result of food, fluid, or stomach contents entering the lungs. It usually occurs in people who have conditions resulting in the loss of their gag or cough reflex. This sometimes happens after a stroke, brain injury, or advanced dementia. Dislodged or misplaced nasogastric tubes are also a cause of aspiration pneumonia. When food and fluids enter the lungs, they irritate and obstruct the delicate airways, introducing millions of microbes into the lung. Aspiration pneumonia is more common in the lower lobe of the right lung as the anatomy of the airways means that solids and liquids are more likely to be inhaled in that direction.

- **'Walking' or 'Atypical' Pneumonia:** Sometimes, people have a milder form of pneumonia and do not become severely ill; they may be able to continue normal activities but feel a little unwell. People may feel that the symptoms are too mild to see a doctor and have a proper diagnosis, and so 'walking' pneumonia may be more common than we realise.

Section 7

Pneumonia Risk Factors

Some people are more at risk than others, and being aware of your risk factors can help you make healthy choices to avoid serious illness. Common risk factors include:

- **Having A Pre-Existing Condition:** Existing health conditions that affect the lungs, such as chronic obstructive pulmonary disease (COPD), asthma, or heart failure can increase the chances of an individual developing pneumonia.

- **A Weakened Immune System:** Some medications, particularly those given for cancer or for autoimmune diseases, disrupt the immune system and make it difficult to fight infections. Some conditions directly affect the immune system, such as AIDS.

- **Age**: Young children and the elderly population are more likely to develop pneumonia and related complications.

- **Smoking:** Smokers are much more likely to develop pneumonia and other lung disorders. Second-hand smoke is just as harmful and children who live in houses where people smoke are more likely to get pneumonia.

- **Dysphagia:** Dysphagia refers to difficulty in swallowing. People with dysphagia often have a reduced gag and cough reflex, meaning that food, fluids, and all kinds of microbes can enter the windpipe and stay in the lungs. Groups who may suffer from dysphagia include people with Parkinson's disease or advanced dementia and individuals who have had a stroke.

- **Spinal Cord Injuries:** Aside from potential swallowing difficulties, people with severe spinal cord injuries may be reliant on mechanical ventilation and have complex tracheostomy (a breathing tube through the front of the throat into the windpipe) care needs. They may also be unable to cough without mechanical assistance and hence find it harder to clear their lungs.

- **A Recent Illness**: Having had a recent illness or being generally run-down and unwell can mean that it's harder to fight off further illnesses.

- **Drinking too much alcohol or using drugs** increases your risk of pneumonia because you may aspirate food, drink, or vomit into your lungs while inebriated.

- **Malnutrition:** It increases the chance of acquiring the condition and making it more severe, particularly in young children and the elderly.

- Poor dental care can also be a cause, especially if you wear dentures.

- Animals, chemicals, or environmental toxins: Being in close proximity to animals might expose you to infected droppings that end up in the soil. Pneumonia can also increase by exposure to certain chemicals and pollution.

Section 8

Diagnosing Pneumonia

Typically, investigations for pneumonia begin when someone presents to their doctor or at a hospital with the symptoms of a chest infection – usually breathlessness, chest pain, coughing, and feeling generally unwell. The doctor will ask about your medical history, particularly risk factors and exposure, and the symptoms you are experiencing.

The doctor will need to listen to the sounds of your breathing so will use a stethoscope held against a few different places on your chest and back. The doctor may also use a pulse oximeter, which is a device that clips onto your fingertip, to measure the amount of oxygen in your blood.

A chest X-ray is one of the best tools used to diagnose and plan treatment for pneumonia, as it enables the doctor to visualize the amount of inflammation and fluids in the lungs, and exactly where they are. An x-ray can also show if there are any larger collections of fluid in or around the lungs. If your cough is 'productive' – if you are coughing up any phlegm – a sample should be taken to try and find out the specific type of microbe causing the infection.

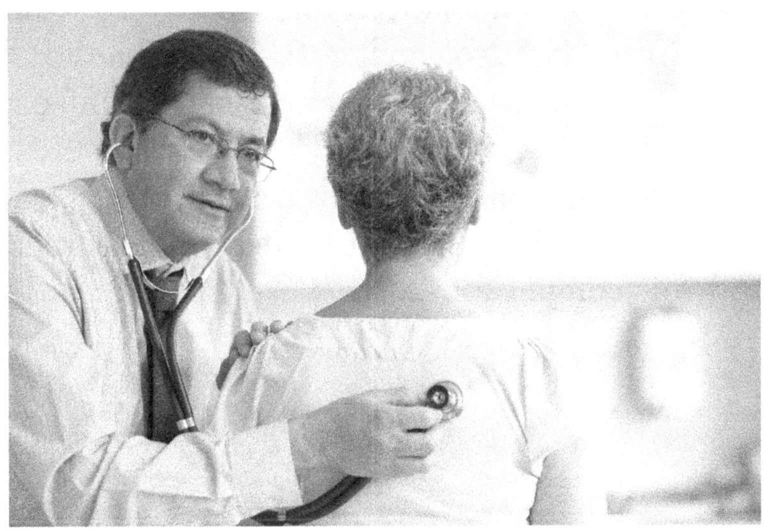

Section 9

Treatment for Pneumonia

Treatment for pneumonia will change depending on the severity of the illness. In most cases, pneumonia can be treated by resting sufficiently. Not only that, antibiotics are prescribed if there is a bacterial infection. Generally, drinking plenty of fluids is a sure way to rejuvenate your body system. The goal of treatment is to cure the infection, in order to avoid complications.

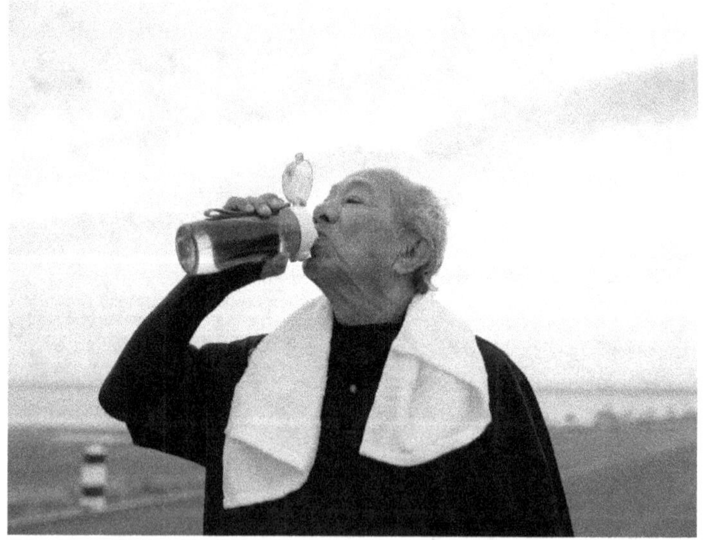

Mild cases of pneumonia, particularly in people without any significant risk factors, may be manageable at home, but should be assessed by a doctor. Seeing a doctor means that they can prescribe antibiotics if they think it is likely to be bacterial pneumonia. Rest, fluids, antibiotics and simple over-the-counter treatments for pain and fever may be enough to treat mild cases of pneumonia.

For more severe cases of pneumonia, with chest pain, breathing difficulties and where the person becomes seriously unwell, a hospital admission will be necessary. Sometimes, people with mild pneumonia but who are at risk of becoming seriously ill and unable to clear the infection at home – people on medication to suppress the immune system, for example – may be admitted to hospital before they become seriously unwell.

In hospital, treatment for pneumonia will most likely take the form of strong intravenous (IV) antibiotics, IV fluids, and possible oxygen through a mask or a tube that sits in the nostrils. Vital signs will also be taken regularly to monitor your progress. This will include measuring your blood pressure, temperature, oxygen levels, heart rate and breathing rate.

Most people are able to manage cough and fever symptoms by the following:

- Medication to bring down the fever
- Drinking fluids in order to loosen and bring up phlegm
- Drinking warm beverages, taking hot baths and using a humidifier to open up the airways for easier breathing
- Avoiding smoke
- Being rested

In some cases, one may be given intravenous fluids and antibiotics, alongside oxygen therapy for assistance.

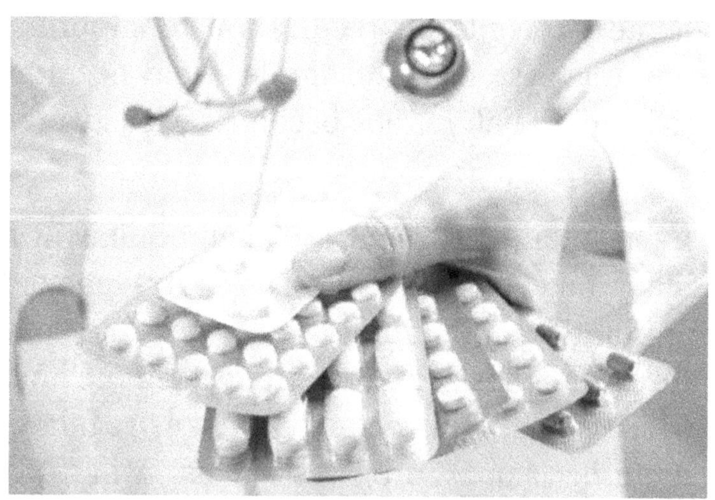

Section 10

Managing Pneumonia

Pneumonia management is different for everyone, depending on the underlying cause and your health condition. Some cases of pneumonia can be managed at home, whereas others will need hospital admission.

- **Managing Pneumonia At Home:** Less severe cases of pneumonia can be managed at home. Maintaining an upright or slightly inclined position can help to keep the lungs clear. If you experience pain and fever, over-the-counter medications can help. A doctor may also prescribe antibiotic tablets if they think it is likely to be a bacterial infection. If you're managing pneumonia at home, it's important to know when to see a doctor or get more urgent help – if you become short of breath, drowsy, or develop severe pain.
- **Managing Pneumonia In Hospitals:** In a hospital, healthcare professionals will closely monitor your temperature,

breathing rate, oxygen levels, heart rate and blood pressure. This helps to guide treatment and identify problems early. People with severe infections may need to be given intravenous (drip) fluids and antibiotics. Blood tests and sputum samples may be taken to make sure any antibiotics are targeting the right types of microbe. Doctors and nurses can also try to identify and manage any underlying cause of this pneumonia, for example, a reduced swallowing ability. Treatment in hospitals means that there are more options for treatment if pneumonia becomes more serious, such as specialist physiotherapists to help with breathing exercises to clear the lungs, non-invasive ventilators, and oxygen therapy.

Section 11

Complications of Pneumonia

Most people, particularly those who are reasonably healthy to start with, recover from pneumonia with no complications. However, pneumonia can be a serious illness and is not always easy to treat. Severe pneumonia can trigger other serious conditions such as:

- **Sepsis:** This is where the body's inflammatory response to infection affects several organ systems. Kidney, heart and lung function may all be reduced. Around 20% of all deaths worldwide are caused by sepsis.

- **Abscesses in the lungs:** A pocket of infected pus could develop in the lung. Larger abscesses may need to be drained.

- **Respiratory failure:** This may occur if the function of the lungs is so reduced that the gas exchange is unable to meet the body's demand. People with respiratory failure can become ill very quickly and need intensive care.

- **Pleural effusion:** Due to the inflammation in the lungs, fluid collects between the pleura and the chest wall. Pleural effusion might lead to the collapse of the lungs if not treated properly.

- **Endocarditis/Pericarditis:** Because blood circulates through the heart muscles and pericardium, there is a greater risk of infection there if bacteremia is present.

- **Septicemia** (Septicemia is the clinical name for blood poisoning by bacteria). It is a medical emergency and needs urgent medical treatment): Because bacteremia can occur in pneumonia, it can lead to septicemia.

Section 12

Preventing Pneumonia

Pneumonia cannot always be prevented, but there are some steps we can take to avoid becoming ill, and to ensure that we're able to recover as quickly and fully as possible when we do become ill. Below are some preventive ways:

- **Vaccination:** Getting vaccinated is the first line of protection against pneumonia. Several vaccinations are available to help prevent pneumonia. Pneumovax 23 and Prevnar 13 These two pneumonia vaccinations assist to protect against pneumococcal pneumonia and meningitis. Your doctor can advise you on which option is best for you. Prevnar 13 works against 13 different kinds of pneumococcal bacteria. For those who have had a bone marrow transplant, Vaccines for pneumonia will not prevent all cases of the disease, according to the National Heart, Lung, and Blood.

- **Quit Smoking:** Stopping smoking is one of the best things you can do for all aspects of your health, and that of the people around you. Smoking directly causes serious lung diseases and impairs the natural defences of the respiratory system.

- **Observe Good Hygiene Standards:** Handwashing, using and promptly throwing away tissues, and avoiding mingling with people who are ill can help to reduce our chances of developing pneumonia. If everyone follows basic hygiene standards, the risks of passing on coughs and colds can be greatly reduced.

- **Stay Healthy:** We can't always avoid catching a cough or chest infection, but if we generally follow a healthy lifestyle to try and maintain a baseline of good health, we're less likely to become seriously unwell.

- **Manage Existing Conditions:** If you have specific risk factors for pneumonia, managing them as well as possible is important. Maintaining good control of conditions like asthma or heart failure, and attending regular chronic disease management appointments can help prevent further complications.

- **Stay Up-To-Date With Vaccinations:** Those at a higher risk of developing pneumonia are recommended to have seasonal vaccines. These include the flu vaccine and pneumococcal vaccine, which protects against a kind of bacteria that commonly causes pneumonia.

- **Staying Well And Getting The Right Care:** The people most at risk of contracting or developing serious complications from pneumonia are usually those who already have other illnesses. Leading a healthy lifestyle, going for regular health screenings and ensuring that you are generally healthy is important.